The

Pilates

Workout

Journal

Also by the authors
The Pilates Powerhouse

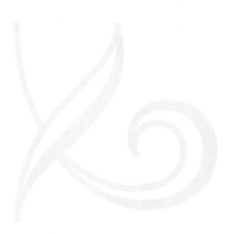

The Pilates Workout Journal

AN **EXERCISE DIARY**
& **CONDITIONING GUIDE**

Mari Winsor with Mark Laska

Perseus Publishing Cambridge, Massachusetts

Printed in the United States of America.

Perseus Publishing is a member of the Perseus Books Group

Text design by mwdesign
Set in Filosofia

First printing, March 2001

Visit us on the World Wide Web at http://www.perseusbooks.com

Perseus books are available at special discounts for bulk purchases in the U.S. by corporations, institutions, and other organizations. For more information, please contact the Special Markets Department at the Perseus Books Group, 11 Cambridge Center, Cambridge, MA 02142, or call (617)252-5298.

1 2 3 4 5 6 7 8 9 10—03 02 01

Contents

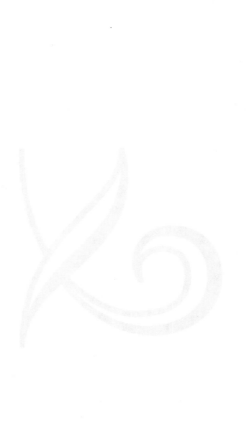

Introduction

Over the years, I have seen wall calendars replaced by desktop appointment books, which were replaced by leather-bound day planners, which have been replaced by palm-sized electronic scheduling devices. With their aid, I have been more efficient at scheduling my day, remembering my appointments, and keeping my work life together. In short, they work, and work well. There are some activities, however, that I want to separate from the rest of my life ... activities that rejuvenate my mind and body ... activities that are designed to take my mind off my hectic schedule, that relax me, that provide a sanctuary. These activities are solely for my peace of mind, my betterment, and to give me perspective on the rest of my busy schedule. For these activities, I prefer a completely different method of cataloging my time — a method that does not muddy the waters of my life's aspirations with details of hair appointments, dog washing, and grocery lists. I need a place where I can explore what I dream to be, and not be distracted by appointments later that day or lists of people I have to call. I need a log that is a clean slate, a journal in which to chart goals, note insights and profound thoughts, and ponder the meaning of life. I need a book that is used for nothing else except to explore the person I wish to become, and to note the progress of the person I am becoming.

Pilates is the most exciting and beneficial form of exercise that I have ever experienced. In using Pilates, I have found that sanctuary, that activity that both improves my appearance and provides inspiration. I have been doing Pilates for over twenty years, and each time I go through the routine, I have an epiphany — about the exercise, or the nuances of the human body, or about life itself.

In my experience, though, these insights can be fleeting. With the intention of holding on to these thoughts, I began keeping a journal that I use with my workouts. In it, I make notations of what exercises I performed and how different parts of my body were feeling. I track my progress, note my personal victories, express the overwhelming feelings of euphoria or stress reduction or overall well-being that are unique to this form of exercise upon completion, and write down the thoughts and insights that come to me in these moments of total clarity. I have found this journal to be one of the most effective tools to both indicate my progress and insure that I never lose those flashes of inspiration and once-in-a-lifetime ideas. In creating The Pilates Workout Journal I have improved upon what I personally use, and have every hope that this will be even more useful for you.

Why should I use
a workout journal?

I was first exposed to Pilates when I began my career as a professional dancer and choreographer. At the height of my professional dancing career I was involved in a serious motorcycle accident. My body was broken and mangled. Any movement was excruciating. After being told that I might never dance again, I began using Pilates to rehabilitate my injuries. Simply getting out of bed was seen as a personal victory. I started using a journal to make notation on which exercises I was using, how my body felt that day. If there were problem areas or challenges in the movement, I tracked my range of motion, how far I could go or how flexible certain body parts were, and my level of strength. By concentrating on positive progress, rather than how much pain I was in, I was able to push myself a little further each day. After two months of this daily practice, I was dancing again.

If you are just beginning this form of exercise, and have been to a class or have seen a video, you may be a little intimidated. Believe me, no one can just start this form of exercise and execute the positions perfectly right off the bat. The people that can perform this exercise flawlessly should be seen as an inspiration. You should not compare yourself to them, but rather be inspired to someday be able to be as accomplished. I can assure you that with a little diligence, you will develop your own potential. There is no other person to compete with when you do Pilates. It is your muscle tone you are improving. It is your flexibility you are concerned with. It is your tummy that is getting more trim and defined. It is your bottom that is becoming firmer. The only competition you will encounter comes from within. You will be inspired to push yourself a little further each day if you can note just how far you came. It takes time. It takes patience. It takes the ability to mark your progress.

Marking your progress is completely subjective. Unlike the long jump, where you can clearly see a measurement, or running a race where you can check your time, Pilates requires that you use other tools to measure just how far you have come. With Pilates we rely on subjective measurements, such as how flexible your muscles were, how strong you felt, your energy level before, during, and after your workout, and how you *feel* after the workout. Pilates is a form of exercise that is as much about your mind as it is about your body. It is about positively enhancing your head-space as much as it is about toning your muscles, and there is no better way to measure reduction of stress, clarity of thought, inner calm and centeredness, than by your own inner barometer. This journal will help you to refine this inner barometer, this inner guide, which I believe can be one of your greatest tools in life.

How to use
The Pilates Workout Journal

P ilates is not a team sport. It is a discipline that is a unique experience for each and every person that is actively engaged in its perfection. Your goal is to have all the different parts of your body working together in unison and harmony to execute each exercise as perfectly as possible at a given moment, and seamlessly link each exercise to the next as one piece of continuous movement. To seek perfection requires dedication. You must be an active participant—you must push yourself in that pursuit of perfection. Whether you are doing Pilates alone in the privacy of your own home, or are working with an instructor, you will have to learn to rely on yourself to measure your own success. In doing so, you will also become the coach of your own team. By using the workout journal you will learn to be the best coach you can be. In becoming the coach of your own body, you will become the master of all you possess.

Using The Pilates Workout Journal couldn't be easier.

First, complete the mat routine of your choice (see the back of this journal for a list of beginner, intermediate, and advanced exercises in the order you should perform them), or finish your workout using the Pilates machines. Then, simply open up the workout journal, find the next unused page and fill in the blanks.

You will see five different headings on each page. These

5

headings all pertain to significant areas that are worthy of reflection. First, write in today's date at the bottom of the page, and then fill out the rest of the page from top to bottom using these suggestions and asking yourself the following questions.

The first space is dedicated to Strength & Flexibility. Write a sentence or two about the way your workout *felt*. Did you feel your energy change during the workout? Were your muscles tight, or did you feel especially limber? Perhaps you would like to add a little more detail. Noting particular exercises, could you get a fuller stretch today? How much further could you go? Were there any parts of the body that felt weaker? Is one arm or one leg stronger than the other? Is one side of your body stronger than the other? Is there a difference in flexibility? Is there a portion of your body that needs to become more limber? Did you remember to "work to the weaker side" during your workout? In the course of today's workout, did you have a breakthrough, or learn a strength and flexibility trick that was the key to a better execution? What is it about your strength or your flexibility that you would like to concentrate on? What are your strength and flexibility goals for your next workout? Did you come upon a long-term goal regarding your strength or flexibility? If so, what is your plan to achieve that goal?

The next space is reserved for Endurance. Pilates is different each day. It can be physically taxing or can completely energize you. Very much like running a race, the goal is of course to cross the finish line, but analyzing each step can be helpful in running a better race the next time. How did you start? What were the first ten minutes of your workout like? Could you get through the routine with verve, or did your energy fall off somewhere? Where did it lag? Where did it speed up? Did you finish with energy? Did you do something differently today that helped power you through a certain segment of the routine? How do feel at this very moment? On a scale of 1 to 10, how would you rate your endurance today?

The space dedicated to Coordination & Balance is for only positive thoughts and notations of progress. In this space I would suggest that you reflect on what went right today. When contemplating your coordination and balance, I want you to concentrate on what went particularly well. What exercises were particularly smooth? Did you achieve a breakthrough today? Where did you feel the most graceful? Where did you achieve a sense of beauty in your movement? What specific aspect of your coordination and your balance improved today? Would you describe your movement as graceful or robotic?

The space reserved for Challenges is just that . . . a challenge. A challenge is not negative or positive. It is just an area that needs concentration. Again I urge you to release any negative thoughts about yourself, the method, or any self-consciousness you experience with the movement. Be objective rather than emotional about these challenges. Even the most advanced Pilates practitioners can find something to improve upon. Even if the challenge seems daunting, you can chip away at it to make it smaller. Where were you challenged today? Where would you like to focus in your next workout? What would you like to improve? As your own coach, what suggestion would you make to yourself the next time you work out?

The last entry on the page is reserved exclusively for Mind & Spirit. This is the area that I sometimes fill out first. I get a flash of brilliance . . . a lightning bolt of an idea . . . a profound insight into life that just cannot wait for reflection. Of course, that doesn't happen every day. In that case, I complete this portion of the page last, and sometimes that insight occurs while I write down my thoughts or experiences. Start by just noting how you feel at this very moment. Like some kind of beautiful drug, completing your Pilates workout can cause a "high" of sorts. Feelings of euphoria, excessive happiness, of being completely energized, and feeling especially vital, are all worth noting. Pilates also offers a world of benefits that you may be feeling at this particular moment. How is your level of stress? How clear is your head? Are you smiling? Does your heart feel open? Do you feel focused? How centered do you feel? How alive does every cell of your body feel at this very moment? I sometimes even add to this entry later on in the day. Over the years I have learned that I can attribute so many positive occurrences to this form of exercise. You may feel better equipped to meet challenges at work. You may be more receptive to friends and loved ones. You may notice a sense of peacefulness in your demeanor. You may have poise under pressure, or find that your level of patience, empathy, or compassion is dramatically improved. Your centeredness may help you to see situations for what they really are. You may have total clarity about your world, your life, your situation, or your surroundings. Your sex life may be improved. Your health may benefit. Nagging injuries or physical ailments may be relieved or healed. Without exception, everyone I train eventually tells me "Pilates changed my life." More and more, you will make notations of how it is changing yours.

Whether you are just beginning this routine or have done it for years, making notes about your progress, or the way you performed today, or what you experienced will enable you to become more proficient in your workout, and eventually to become a master of this method of body conditioning. Over time, I have discovered that most of the thoughts in my personal journal were concentrated in these five areas. When combined, these areas of concentration are the foundation for bringing a sense of quality to your Pilates workout. When there is quality in your workout, you will experience an amazing new inner world of understanding, and be the recipient of a host of benefits that are unique to this form of exercise.

The evolution of Pilates

Pilates (Pil-Ah-Tees) is a form of exercise named after its inventor. Joseph Pilates was a revolutionary force in the world of fitness. Amazingly, he invented this scientific system of body conditioning over eighty years ago, and after decades of research, compiled these findings to create the form of exercise that is so wildly popular to this day. As we begin the new millennium, Pilates exercise has established itself as both a concept whose time has come, and the most practical application of an exercise that blends East and West. Pilates represents the total mind/body experience that can be effortlessly fit into our hectic schedules.

Joseph Pilates was born in Germany in 1880. He was a frail child with serious health problems. As a young man, he became passionate about physical fitness as a way to transform his physical appearance and improve his health. As he grew older, he became an accomplished gymnast, boxer, and circus performer, and was also an ardent student of Eastern philosophies such as yoga and karate. He called upon all of his research, study and expertise to create a complete regimen that combined East and West, gymnastic and yogic principles, mental and physical exercises that would strengthen the body and free the mind.

Word of Pilates' remarkable conditioning system spread throughout Germany. The Kaiser demanded that Pilates use his method to train his elite troops. As he was an ardent pacifist, he politely declined, and moved to England to take a job in the circus. Just as he was reaching the peak of his career as a performer, World War I broke out and he was interred for the duration of the war.

As you may well imagine, a prison camp is most certainly the worst possible environment to maintain a healthy body, let alone a healthy spirit. Pilates, however, somehow grew stronger in these surroundings. He employed all of his knowledge to create a method of body conditioning that helped him to survive. He became very resourceful, and utilized any resource available to him. When people are first introduced to Pilates, they are introduced to an intimidating array of machines and devices. Joseph Pilates fashioned these machines from anything that was readily available, his bunk, the bedsprings, and his famous chair, and an entire routine that required no equipment at all that is referred to as the mat routine.

His fellow prisoners knew that he had discovered something miraculous. He began to teach this method of body conditioning to them, and to their delight, they began to thrive. Soon after, he began teaching his method to the prison guards. They found this method so successful that it became a mandatory activity for the entire camp.

For prisoners and guards alike, remaining healthy in these camps was an even larger concern than physical fitness. Disease was a major concern. As the most brutal war man had ever known was nearing an end, the influenza epidemic of 1918 spread across the globe. It is estimated that four million lives were lost as a result of World War I. It is estimated that the flu epidemic of 1918 claimed over fifty million lives. In rural towns, it was not unusual that 70 percent of the population died from this epidemic. In urban or confined areas, where the disease could be spread much more rapidly, these numbers were even greater. It is remarkable that not *one* internee in the camp died from the epidemic, and Pilates himself always attributed that amazing statistic to his method. This did not escape the attention of the British military establishment. It was not long after that Pilates was employed to train the most elite cadre of British troops.

Joseph Pilates' fame grew during this period just after the war, and many performers and athletes turned to him for training. Among the many who sought his talent was the heavyweight boxing phenomenon, Max Schmelling. As Pilates was an accomplished boxer himself, he was able to lend not only his expertise and knowledge of the sport but also his revolutionary method of conditioning to Schmelling's camp. Schmelling became so enamored of Pilates that the two became inseparable friends. As Schmelling worked his way up the ranks, he was given a shot at a championship title fight in New York City. The financial opportunities for professional athletes were much more plentiful there, and Schmelling decided that it would be advantageous to emigrate. This move meant that it would be necessary to bring all of his promotional, business, and training staff with him. By this time Pilates was a close confidant and a valuable member of his entourage, but was reticent to follow. Desperate for his participation, Schmelling's manager agreed to finance a studio in New York, as a bonus of sorts for Pilates.

Pilates left his adopted England for a new land, a new start, and a new life. On his journey he met the woman who would soon be his wife. With her help and the backing of Schmelling's manager, Pilates set up his first legitimate studio on Eighth Avenue in New York City. In almost no time the studio attracted an eclectic and influential following. It seemed that the most famous and interesting people in the world made Pilates' studio their home away from home. Among the many devoted subscribers to his method were Ruth St. Denis and Ted Shawn, perhaps the most celebrated names in dance at the time. Through their introduction, Pilates soon took on as students Martha Graham and George Balanchine, the founders of modern dance. Graham and Balanchine became early pioneers of the method. Balanchine went so far as to incorporate, move for move, Pilates' mat routine into one of his most famous dance pieces, "Seven Deadly Sins."

During this period, my mentor, Romana Kryzanowska, was introduced to Pilates by George Balanchine, and began studying the Pilates method. She is now in her seventies, and because she has meant so much to me and this work, I have added some of her experiences so that you can see firsthand how this method has been passed from generation to generation. "When I was first introduced to Joseph Pilates," states Romana, "I had injured my ankle quite badly and was not able to dance. Back then there was no such thing as physical therapy or sports medicine, and the only alternative was surgery, and even that was primitive. Joe said, 'This is how it works, you sign up for five lessons, and if your ankle is not better I will refund your money.'" Romana decided to give this man a chance. "My first lesson," Romana explains, "I thought this man was crazy. He had me doing exercises that were not specific to my ankle. How could this help me? After all I was a professional dancer that could do all these marvelous things with my body. The last thing I felt I needed was more exercise." Throughout her first lesson she continued to ask what these exercises were for and why she needed to do them. After her third lesson, she noticed that there was no swelling in her ankle, and that she no longer felt any pain. It was then she learned the first principle of this work: "Circulation is what heals."

After this third lesson, she returned to ballet class. "I noticed something that was different, an extreme, in tune, sense of balance and strength that I did not have before working with Joe. I noticed an utter control, and felt that I was master over every body part, and it would move wherever I wanted it to go. My leg was perfect and my work was better than it ever was. I have believed in Pilates ever since." She became so intrigued that she spent much time with Joseph Pilates. "He knew the inner workings of the body so well, and understood the dynamics of the inner world that we are just becoming aware of today. He was an almost magical man, perhaps the most remarkable healer I have ever witnessed, who also had a very keen mind. He read constantly, and his studies of mathematics and laws of physics are directly related to every single exercise in this method."

After the death of Joseph Pilates in the late 1960s, Romana single-handedly kept this form alive. The evolution of this form has been altered slightly as a new generation of professionals have come to the work and added an exercise here or there to develop different parts of the body. The integrity of this work was preserved by Sean Gallagher, who founded Performing Art Physical Therapy/The Pilates Studio of New York. Along with experts such as Romana Kryzanowska, he is responsible for the certification of teachers, and the methods employed to instruct. As both a certified Pilates instructor and a practicing physical therapist, Gallagher has truly incorporated and integrated Pilates into modalities of treatment that health care practitioners can provide and utilize.

I first was introduced to this work in the context of dance. The methodology was easily incorporated into the techniques and principles I had learned throughout my life as a professional. Originally, I had come to the work to offset the physical demands of my chosen field. At a time when I should have been considering retirement, I found that my body was getting much stronger, that nagging injuries and soreness no longer hampered me, and that my overall health was much improved. My lifelong asthma problems were significantly decreased through the utilization of Pilates techniques, and I found myself better equipped in my professional life. After only one class with the woman who would become my mentor, I became a student of Romana Kryzanowska, and increased my understanding and respect for this work. As my understanding deepened, my professional career improved, and because of this work, I was able to dance professionally until I reached the age of forty. The work became so inspiring that I began to subsidize my income by teaching the Pilates technique. Teaching the technique, especially the profound mental and spiritual benefits Pilates offers, became so rewarding that I dedicated my life to passing this knowledge to others.

It has been my honor to teach this method of body conditioning to literally thousands of people. In 1990, I opened Winsor Fitness in Los Angeles. The studio was an instant success, and attracted dozens of high-profile clientele. I have trained many celebrities and professional athletes. To them, and to their dedication to this work, I am deeply and profoundly indebted. Their dedication to this work helped them change their lives dramatically. Those physical and mental changes became so significant in their lives that they began speaking publicly about it. Over the last decade, some of my high-profile clientele have endorsed their work with me in the media, and this has significantly elevated the work in the public's awareness. This awareness has risen to such a degree that Pilates has become the "in" thing to do, and has reached almost fad-like popularity. The intense demand for this work, along with my great friend Danny Glover, enabled me to open a second studio for Los Angeles' West Side, Winsor West. Still, I could not meet the high demand for this knowledge, and was approached to write The Pilates Powerhouse and this companion workout journal, so that you, the reader, could benefit from this incredible method of body conditioning.

Pilates has completely changed my life. It enabled me to dance professionally until I was forty, it has helped keep debilitating asthma at bay so that I am able to maintain a healthy lifestyle, it has helped me recover from devastating injury, it has transformed my self-image and sense of worth, and on a daily basis it keeps me calm and centered. It is my greatest hope in bringing this work to you, that if I can pass on even a small morsel of the infinite benefits this routine offers, in some small way I will improve the quality of life for those that read this. It is my honor to be a link in the long lineage of teachers who have brought this information into our collective consciousness.

Principles of understanding
& the science of the art

To experience what I refer to as the *Joy of Movement*, or to derive the full benefit that this method of body conditioning offers, it is important to be aware that there are certain scientific principles at work. Some learn these principles in a logical linear fashion, some absorb meaning on a more ethereal or conceptual level, and others learn by way of the body informing them — from the practice of performing the exercise. In whatever manner you derive understanding, it is important that you know the fundamentals of Pilates.

The principles of this exercise are easy enough to comprehend. Basically, it is a series of exercises or poses that are connected to scientifically strengthen a specific area of the body. As a whole, the routine brings the body into a state of harmony, so that all these areas are working together as one unit. Unlike most exercise, it is not how much, how strong, and how many, but rather it is a sense of the whole body working in unison that is the goal.

You are to be *present* for this exercise. Don't leave your brain in the locker room. Yes, you will be performing a very specific routine; however, it is the elements that you bring to that routine that make this method valuable. As I stated in the last chapter, you are creating a certain level of quality in your life by partaking in this form of exercise, and to achieve that quality requires your full participation. There are tools that you bring to the physical work of this exercise that will help you to derive the even greater benefits of the work. Namely, the tools you will need to have in your workshop are breathing, relaxation, concentration, control, and a heightened sense of fluidity.

BREATHING

Breathing is a bodily function that we perform whether we are conscious of it or not. The trick is to be very mindful of the manner in which we are breathing. In this form of exercise, each movement is tied to a specific manner of breathing. The breath allows oxygen to nourish the muscles being utilized, and to release an array of non-beneficial chemicals stored in the muscles. These chemicals are related to pain and fatigue, and they are substances that we are desperately trying to rid ourselves of. To do this requires not only that we take in an ample supply of oxygen, but also that we are fully and purposefully exhaling, or what I call wringing out the lungs.

Different disciplines require different methods of breathing. For instance, an opera singer breathes air in below the diaphragm, puffing the stomach out. A musician, especially a woodwind or brass player, breathes into the stomach, and proceeds to fill the entire chest cavity and then the throat with air. For this specific form of exercise, it is entirely possible that you will have to retrain yourself to breathe in a new way. When most of us inhale, we expand the top of our chest. We may think that this is a deep breath, but truly, it is shallow breathing. An extreme example of this is when an asthmatic has an attack. Breathing becomes very labored, and air is gasped into only the uppermost portion of the lungs, in an action that more resembles swallowing than breathing. Instead, what we need to learn is to breathe into the back in the area that expands the small ribs. In other words, rather than having our breath expand the front of our chest outwards or puff our stomach out, we concentrate on filling the bottommost portion of our lungs, and get the sensation that we are breathing into the small of our back. This form of deep breathing allows us to bend and move without restricting the amount of oxygen that we are taking in. The oxygen intake allows nourishment to travel to the muscles being worked. As we fully exhale, it allows all of the unused gasses and non-beneficial chemicals stored within the body a route of escape. When we expel these elements, we become more clear-headed, our stamina increases, we release lactic acids within the musculature that make us feel sore, and most importantly, we become more relaxed.

RELAXATION

One of the skills you will need to learn immediately is how to work out without creating undue tension in areas of the body that are not being worked. When people first begin this work, they are simply working too hard. Some people, especially men, have been exercising in a manner that requires brute strength, and oftentimes it is the effort put forth that lends the best end result. In Pilates, just the opposite is true. You will be working a specific area of the body in each separate exercise (believe me, you will know where it is) and as those specific areas are being worked, it is your task to make certain that the areas not involved are working to support the movement. When you are riding a horse, there is more to steering than merely sitting on top of the animal, and leaving it up to the discretion of the horse to stay on the trail or not.

You are holding the reins, your shoulders are relaxed but ready, your feet are flexed in the stirrups waiting to signal, and you are squeezing with your legs. Your whole body is involved. With Pilates, it is the involvement of the entire body that helps to relieve tension in the body. After you finish the routine you will notice that you have eliminated stress significantly on both the physical and mental levels.

CONCENTRATION

As our ability to concentrate on a specific area of the body improves, we dramatically enhance the quality of our movement. The movements you will be executing are very specific to an area of the body, and it is essential that you concentrate your attention to insure that that specific area is working correctly. Often when we move, we are completely unconscious. The brain gets an image of what we want to do, and without really paying attention, the body executes what the brain intended. For instance, there is a significant distinction between lifting up a glass that has been filled to the brim, and when, as you read the morning paper, you reach for your cup of coffee without looking. When a brain surgeon is working, you can be fairly certain that any movement that surgeon makes is deliberate and intentional. When we are mindful of our movement, we can employ both the brain and the body to work harmoniously and effectively. Throughout the exercise portion of the book, I will not only provide you areas of the body that you are concentrating on moving, but will give you some helpful imagery as well.

CONTROL

Control is an essential key to the quality of your movement. This is not an overly exertive form of exercise; it is specific and intentional movement. You will not be flailing your limbs here and there, you will be moving with the grace of a dancer, having several parts of the body engaged in mindful movement simultaneously. There are never movements that are propelled by the momentum of throwing a part of the body. The exercise is instead initiated by a stretch, and completed by way of contraction or force. When you first begin this method of body conditioning, you may go through an awkward stage. The exercises could involve parts of the body that you are not used to moving in unison. Have no fear, once you have the basic understanding of the move, you will be able to execute the movements gracefully.

FLUIDITY

The quality of being graceful while you perform this movement stems from the fluidity of one movement seamlessly blending into the next. I think of this whole exercise as being a perfectly choreographed dance piece, and to perform it with grace means to execute the movements with that precision. Each movement or exercise has a specific point at which it begins, and a place where it ends. However, it is your task for those places to blend into each other, and to be unrecognizable points of reference within the whole. Even if you may be instructed to hold at a certain point in each movement for a certain number of counts, that hold is not a place to stop, but rather a place where a stretch or movement continues, however unrecognizable it may be to an outside observer. Each exercise leads to the next. There is really no time when the movement stops ... The end of one movement is just the beginning of another.

Conceptually, Pilates is an exercise that is paradoxical, or based on premises that may seem to be diametrically opposed. You will be working from the inside out, and simultaneously working from the outside in. You will be strengthening smaller muscle groups to support the movement and abilities of the larger muscles. You will be moving in a very controlled fashion to free your mind. You will be using your mind to move the body, and when you are finished with this routine, there will be a closer bond between these two aspects of your persona. You will feel whole ... energized ... powerful.

INSIDE OUT / OUTSIDE IN

When done correctly, you will be using your center, or powerhouse — your "inside" — to be the root of all movement. (This region of the body is so fundamental to the work that we will discuss it in detail in the following chapter.) This center is the place that connects the abdominal muscles with the small of the back with the buttocks. From the strength of your powerhouse will emanate dramatic changes in the way you stand, move, walk, carry yourself, and physically relate to the world around you. You will simultaneously be doing an external movement that will vastly improve your inner life. It will positively affect your mental clarity, the way you feel, your confidence level, your energy level, and will also create a sense of tranquility and peace of mind.

STRENGTH & FLEXIBILITY

This work is a combination of art and science. Like a perfectly choreographed dance piece, each movement fluidly melds into the next. Each exercise links breathing with strengthening and stretching. Each movement is designed to scientifically oxygenate, then stretch, then strengthen, and then restretch a particular muscle group. The premise of the work is to strengthen smaller muscle groups to support larger muscles. I'll give you an example. When you pick up a barbell to do a set of curls, the object is to isolate only that muscle, and work it to exhaustion. Pilates actually develops smaller muscles that would go unnoticed with this exercise. Imagine yourself doing that same curl with the same weight in your hand — only do it just a little bit more slowly and with control. You would initiate the motion of your arm from your powerhouse, and you could now feel that same exercise affect your forearm, the shoulder, the scapula, the back and buttocks, while you used your stomach to support the movement. When performed in this manner, all of those muscles are now working in conjunction and harmony with one another to perform the task. Your body is now working together as a unit. The idea is to achieve your potential results more quickly, and without injury, by using all of the tools available to you.

FREEDOM & CONTROL

To hold up that spine properly, you have to strengthen your abdominal musculature. As we focus on pulling in the powerhouse, the place in our gut that links the stomach with the lower back with the butt, we can instantly feel a lengthening sensation in the lower back. If we pull the lateral muscles in the back down, the shoulders drop, the neck lengthens, and the spine becomes straighter. The more we concentrate on these body parts working in harmony with one another, the straighter our spine becomes. Remember the first time someone said, "Sit up straight"? We most probably jutted out our chest. This actually arches the middle of your back. The key is to pull inward into the spine by using your powerhouse. There. Now your spine is supported. If you can learn to control this abdominal region of the body, and initiate movement from this place, a whole new world of physical movement will be revealed to you. This requires intense concentration.

If you can maintain your concentration, and be mindful of the manner in which you are moving, you can experience a peace of mind that is the ultimate freeing experience. To accomplish this you should visualize your body being in cement that is almost dry. This cement does not bind you, and it does not inhibit your breathing, but you have to exert control in order to move. Your movements must not be quick, sporadic, or fast. You must, at all times, maintain control.

Pilates is a series of controlled movements done within the frame of your body, so that any movement will not pull you from the center of your body. So you're always in the frame of your body. You maintain motion within the parameters that are marked by the width of the shoulders and hips. You never move your leg out further than where your shoulder ends. If you're lying on your side, you kick your leg forward and back, but you never take it higher than where your hip is. If you exceed these boundaries, you are inviting injury. Get your ligaments and your smaller muscles stronger. Don't rely solely upon the large muscles to lift your leg up, because inevitably you will injure the smaller muscles that support that movement. Initiate all movement from your powerhouse.

With this exercise there is a routine or structure that will take you through each muscle group. The movements are slow and fluid. This demands that the movements be precise. The precision that this requires will demand physical control from your body. Like Tai Chi Chuan, the movements are not jerky, but rather very fluid. The movements alternate between stretching and strengthening, while breathing deeply into each pose. Like yoga, the combination of breathing, stretching and exerting strength has a very soothing effect. Unlike yoga, the routine is much more active and non-repetitive, and is a routine that can be performed without a sense of boredom. The physical demands of the routine will enable you to feel a very deep sense of relaxation and have a tangible sense that your daily stress is slipping away effortlessly. It is the precise control that you will demand of your body that will magically free your mind up.

You may experience a renewed creativity, and find that spontaneous images may pass through your mind while you perform that physical task. You may process through the nuances of your day, give birth to that really great idea, the pieces to the puzzle may all fall into place . . . Who knows? The only thing I am certain of is this: while you are engaged in this fluid series of physically demanding exercises, your mind will be free to wander wherever it wants to. This is precisely the mind/body connection that you are striving to achieve. This doesn't happen by way of a divine source of inspiration. It occurs by way of a mindful intention to move the body in very specific ways.

The Powerhouse

"The most fundamental and essential ingredient
to perform this routine is The Powerhouse."

The powerhouse is located in the center of the body. It is the exact point between the upper half of your body and the lower half of your body, the place between the right side and left side. Anatomically and scientifically, the powerhouse connects several large groups of muscles. The powerhouse refers to musculature located deep within the abdominal region of the body. It is the place that connects the abdomen with the lower back with the buttocks. Joseph Pilates referred to this area as "the girdle of strength." Scientifically, these muscles are called the *rectus abdominis*, and refer to the oblique muscles, and the *transversus abdominis*. When you see someone with highly developed abdominal musculature, or "the six-pack" as bodybuilders call it, you are looking at these muscles. The exact musculature we refer to as the powerhouse is located beneath these muscles, deeper within the abdomen, and is called the *transversus abdominis*. This muscle group, in association and conjunction with the *multifidus* muscle, is the anchor for the *erector spinae* group. It is at the place where these three muscle groups (the *transversus abdominis*, the *multifidus*, and the *erector spinae*) connect that you find The Powerhouse.

In Pilates, all movements are generated by your powerhouse. This is where all of the energy that you exert comes from. Whenever you do an exercise, movement and control over that movement is always initiated by breathing into and pushing from the powerhouse. Always. This allows blood to flow more freely to the body and to the muscles that you need to work. Most of us who are unhappy with our appearance want to transform this exact area of the body. We want a flatter tummy, and a tighter butt. Engaging in this work will absolutely and positively effect those changes by strengthening the powerhouse. Throughout the routine, there is almost constant initiation and use of the powerhouse, and as a result, this area will become much stronger and will help to reduce injuries. For instance, if there's an exercise that requires me to move from my hips, I have to push into my stomach and initiate the movement from my powerhouse to move my hips. Otherwise, my hips take on the task of moving my entire body, and I can lock up and possibly injure myself. Pilates is the only form of exercise that I am aware of that focuses on strengthening this particular region of the body.

Abdominal muscles crisscross in layers across the front of our bodies like a corset to act as a support for the spine. It is from within the abdominal region of the body, or powerhouse, that we support the spine and all of our major organs. Therefore, when we can strengthen this area, we also dramatically improve our alignment and posture, we can reduce or eliminate many of the problems associated with chronic pain, we can relieve and even reverse conditions that foster back and neck problems, and we may even enhance our overall health.

If your powerhouse is really strong, you can almost always eliminate lower back pain. A lot of people have lower back pain because their center is not strong and they do not understand how to engage and utilize it. When they attempt to pick up a heavy object, or partake in another strenuous activity, they will not utilize their powerhouse to initiate that task. As we strengthen the powerhouse, the bone structure of the body tends to be able to more fully support the weight of the body, and is better prepared to move, to exert itself, and to lift heavy objects. These improvements to the posture will not only help to relieve pain, but will increase your physical and emotional potential. You will learn that you can rely on this routine to mentally and physically condition yourself. From that center, you can control your own transformation.

It is from the reliance upon and strengthening of the powerhouse that you will derive *all* of the physical, mental, and spiritual benefits of this form of exercise.

The powerhouse is key to your physical transformation, but it is also essential in developing a higher, more enlightened self. Physically, the area of the body that I have described as the powerhouse was essential to the evolution of our species. The entire development of man required strength in the abdominal musculature to walk upright. It is precisely this area of our anatomical muscular structure that allows us to stand erect. In standing erect, man went through a process of mental transformation as well. Perhaps the missing link is really not missing at all. Perhaps it is within us. Perhaps when man began to walk, there was new information that he was able to process, or more tools he was able to process that information with. Certainly when children begin to walk, it marks a distinct stage of learning. Is it possible that the powerhouse is another communication center for the body? Of course we have large brains, and this enables us to think and process information, but we receive other information as well. We have the senses, we have instinct, we have intuition and perception, we have feelings . . . information that comes to us on a non-intellectual level. This information comes to us by way of the powerhouse. When we combine the mental and physical sources of information, we as human beings have the unique gift to understand and appreciate our surroundings more fully. The combination of physical and mental information processing just may be the reason why we have cognitive ability to reason, to emote, to express the profundities of our experience, to ponder the mysteries of our surroundings, and perhaps *why* we are the most intelligent form of life on our planet.

When the strength of the powerhouse can adequately support the spine, we begin to strike a balance physically. Along with physical balance, we reap the rewards of balance in many other areas of our life. To achieve balance is to strike a center point. This chapter is specifically about the powerhouse, the exact area of the body that is the center. Much of this work is about finding your center . . . your powerhouse . . . a place of balance. This is a real and tangible place that you will become much more attached to as you participate and grow within this work. A potter would begin by centering the clay on the wheel, before they could successfully create a useful object. A washing machine, if it is off-center, will shake itself into a malfunction and turn itself off. When you are playing sports, you can be put off-balance if you are not centered, and so it is with this work. Scientifically, and physiologically, it stands to reason that anything operates better when it's operated from its center. So it is with your body and in your life. Pilates will allow you to develop that center.

The all-important task is to find your center, or power-house. The notion of being centered is really to combine the physical and mental processes. Often there is a distinction between mind and body. Our goal is to have the mental and physical working in conjunction with one another — a mind/body connection. The brain is the center of all neurological activity, and the seat of our intellectual knowledge. The pow-erhouse is the communication center for the body. Being centered, or striking a balance between the mind and the body, is a place that we want to occupy more and more fre-quently. It is much like a muscle that we want to develop. Be-ing centered helps us to be emotionally available, to be men-tally clear, to be capable of accepting challenges, to become more intuitive and perceptive, and able to achieve our po-tential.

Emotionally, that center is the place where we operate best from. That center is the "us" that we love about our-selves. It is the person that we wish to be all of the time. That center or powerhouse is the place where you speak from. It is where you feel emotional pain. It is where you feel joy and elation. Emotionally, everything hits you there before your brain has a chance to process the information. Whether it is having a conversation that you don't want to have, that con-versation where "You're fired" or "You can't do that thing that you do," it is the powerhouse that is always leading the dance. The information will eventually transfer up to the brain, and you have to force the brain to get the powerhouse to relax, and more and more frequently this will become a winning battle. The more centered I am, the more I pay at-tention to what's happening to my powerhouse, the better my posture is, the more capable I am in every aspect of my daily life.

Mentally, the control that you exert over your powerhouse translates into a calm and clarity, from which you can take life's challenges and deal with them appropriately. We are constantly bombarded by negative stimuli. People project their personal baggage onto us, people can be manipulative, and pull us in different directions. When this happens too frequently, we lose focus. When we are centered mentally, we have the strength to stand up for ourselves, because we are dealing from the truest and purest portion of our being.

As you get more in touch with this physical center, you will become more intuitive. When people say, "I have a gut feeling," they are really not off the mark. This center that you are strengthening allows new information to come in. It is the resting-place of instinct. As you develop this area, you will come to trust this more. You will listen to that little voice that is trying to guide you more frequently. I have learned that this voice informs daily, and all I need to do is be quiet enough in my center to hear it.

As you strengthen your powerhouse, you will, in fact, strengthen every aspect of your life.

It allows for possibility to enter into your mind and your spirit and your life. People say that when they really get into Pilates, it changes their lives completely. Better things come to them. They have greater expectations. They are motivated to do things that they want to do. They are true to their ideals. They can express themselves more honestly. They are more effective at communicating and in their professions. They have fuller, more satisfying personal relationships. The beauty of this form of exercise is that each segment is intended to strengthen this area. Each time you perform this routine, a new element will be revealed to you, and as a result, Pilates will never become boring or repetitive. If this routine becomes your exercise of choice, you will look upon it not as a workout, but as a lifestyle that will continually transform the physical, mental, emotional and spiritual aspects of your life. When you can find your center, and learn to control it, this work, and really everything else in your life, will become much easier to handle.

The

Journal

No matter how uncoor-
dinated you might think
you are, or how insecure
about your body you
think you are . . . all of
that is about to change.

STRENGTH
& FLEXIBILITY

ENDURANCE

COORDINATION
& BALANCE

CHALLENGES

MIND & SPIRIT

DATE

STRENGTH
& FLEXIBILITY

ENDURANCE

COORDINATION
& BALANCE

If Pilates becomes your
exercise of choice, you
will look upon it not
as a workout, but as
a movement that con-
tinually transforms the
physical, mental, emo-
tional and spiritual
aspects of your life.

CHALLENGES

MIND & SPIRIT

DATE

STRENGTH
& FLEXIBILITY

ENDURANCE

COORDINATION
& BALANCE

CHALLENGES

MIND & SPIRIT

DATE

STRENGTH & FLEXIBILITY

ENDURANCE

Doing Pilates, and
doing it properly, is
about going someplace
that you've never gone
before in exercise.
Doing Pilates properly
is about awareness.

COORDINATION & BALANCE

CHALLENGES

MIND & SPIRIT

DATE

In doing Pilates,
you will become
aware that whatever
your body needs most
you will feel first.

STRENGTH
& FLEXIBILITY

ENDURANCE

COORDINATION
& BALANCE

CHALLENGES

MIND & SPIRIT

DATE

STRENGTH & FLEXIBILITY

ENDURANCE

COORDINATION & BALANCE

Each time you perform
your routine, a new
element will be revealed
to you, and as a result,
Pilates will never become
boring or repetitive.

CHALLENGES

MIND & SPIRIT

DATE

When doing Pilates, frequently remind yourself of the importance of the powerhouse. It is from this place that all movement and control should be initiated.

STRENGTH & FLEXIBILITY

ENDURANCE

COORDINATION & BALANCE

CHALLENGES

MIND & SPIRIT

DATE

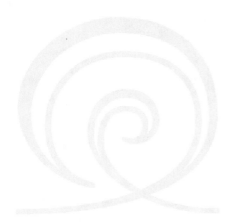

STRENGTH & FLEXIBILITY

ENDURANCE

COORDINATION & BALANCE

"With Pilates you
don't build bulk;
you streamline your
muscles in a way you
can't with any other
form of exercise."
Vanessa Williams

CHALLENGES

MIND & SPIRIT

DATE

STRENGTH
& FLEXIBILITY

ENDURANCE

COORDINATION
& BALANCE

CHALLENGES

MIND & SPIRIT

DATE

Underneath the sternum lies the uppermost portion of the abdominal musculature, and it is this vital area that is largely responsible for maintaining tension within the powerhouse, as well as being the key to your mastery over the control of movement.

The elongation of the
spine is vital in doing
this work correctly, and
holds the key to many
of this routine's great
benefits. Lengthening
your spine is the key to
transforming the way
you look and feel.

STRENGTH
& FLEXIBILITY

ENDURANCE

COORDINATION
& BALANCE

CHALLENGES

MIND & SPIRIT

DATE

MIND & SPIRIT

CHALLENGES

COORDINATION
& BALANCE

ENDURANCE

STRENGTH
& FLEXIBILITY

DATE

STRENGTH
& FLEXIBILITY

ENDURANCE

COORDINATION
& BALANCE

CHALLENGES

MIND & SPIRIT

DATE

STRENGTH & FLEXIBILITY

ENDURANCE

COORDINATION & BALANCE

CHALLENGES

MIND & SPIRIT

I think of Pilates as a ballet. Every movement leads into the next. My routines are scientifically engineered pieces of choreography, to work one specific part of your body after the next. Everything is connected.

DATE

STRENGTH & FLEXIBILITY

ENDURANCE

COORDINATION & BALANCE

CHALLENGES

When you begin to
understand how one
move blends into the
next, you can begin to
concentrate on the
tempo of the routine
as a whole. In Pilates,
there should be no
jerky movements.

MIND & SPIRIT

DATE

If you can maintain your concentration, and be mindful of the manner in which you are moving, you can experience a peace of mind that is the ultimate freeing experience.

STRENGTH
& FLEXIBILITY

ENDURANCE

COORDINATION
& BALANCE

CHALLENGES

MIND & SPIRIT

DATE

STRENGTH
& FLEXIBILITY

ENDURANCE

As you begin Pilates,
you will be keenly aware
of the parts of your body
that are weak and need
to become more flexible.
Gradually, you will notice
a vast improvement in
your overall sense of well
being. You will feel an
almost spiritual connec-
tion to your body.

COORDINATION
& BALANCE

CHALLENGES

MIND & SPIRIT

DATE

STRENGTH
& FLEXIBILITY

ENDURANCE

COORDINATION
& BALANCE

Pilates teaches you to
accept yourself and love
yourself. Only then can
you really change and
transform your body.
You need to find the
joy of moving. Then you
can find the joy of you.

CHALLENGES

MIND & SPIRIT

DATE

STRENGTH
& FLEXIBILITY

ENDURANCE

COORDINATION
& BALANCE

CHALLENGES

MIND & SPIRIT

DATE _____

STRENGTH
& FLEXIBILITY

ENDURANCE

COORDINATION
& BALANCE

CHALLENGES

MIND & SPIRIT

DATE

STRENGTH
& FLEXIBILITY

ENDURANCE

Instead of being a
mindless exercise,
Pilates is very mind-full.
In doing Pilates, you must
concentrate on what
you are doing physically.

COORDINATION
& BALANCE

CHALLENGES

MIND & SPIRIT

DATE

With movement, it is our brain that holds us back, not our bodies. It is our insecurities and thoughts of limitation that truly control our physical limits and performance levels.

STRENGTH & FLEXIBILITY

ENDURANCE

COORDINATION & BALANCE

CHALLENGES

MIND & SPIRIT

DATE

STRENGTH
& FLEXIBILITY

ENDURANCE

COORDINATION
& BALANCE

CHALLENGES

"Pilates gives me
long, lean muscles
and works deeper
than any other work-
outs I've ever done."
Marisa Tomei

MIND & SPIRIT

DATE

MIND & SPIRIT

CHALLENGES

COORDINATION
& BALANCE

ENDURANCE

STRENGTH
& FLEXIBILITY

DATE

STRENGTH & FLEXIBILITY

ENDURANCE

COORDINATION & BALANCE

CHALLENGES

MIND & SPIRIT

There can be no question that Pilates can help us physically, but it is the mental benefits that we receive from this work that can be truly miraculous.

The brain is the center of all neurological activity, and the seat of our intellectual knowledge. The powerhouse is the communication center for the body.

STRENGTH & FLEXIBILITY

ENDURANCE

COORDINATION & BALANCE

CHALLENGES

MIND & SPIRIT

DATE

STRENGTH
& FLEXIBILITY

ENDURANCE

COORDINATION
& BALANCE

Although it is very
simple and will come
to you effortlessly and
unconsciously, the
mental aspect to this
exercise will have pro-
found ramifications for
you throughout your
personal life.

CHALLENGES

MIND & SPIRIT

DATE

MIND & SPIRIT | CHALLENGES | COORDINATION & BALANCE | ENDURANCE | STRENGTH & FLEXIBILITY

DATE

STRENGTH
& FLEXIBILITY

ENDURANCE

COORDINATION
& BALANCE

CHALLENGES

MIND & SPIRIT

When you begin this
exercise routine, you
will immediately feel
your weakest areas.
So what? So you have a
weak area . . . Get over it.
We all have them!

DATE

STRENGTH & FLEXIBILITY

ENDURANCE

COORDINATION & BALANCE

CHALLENGES

Pilates is a series of
controlled movements
done within the frame
of your body, so that
any movement will not
pull you from the center
of your body.

MIND & SPIRIT

DATE

STRENGTH
& FLEXIBILITY

ENDURANCE

COORDINATION
& BALANCE

CHALLENGES

MIND & SPIRIT

The first step to doing
Pilates is accepting where
you are at right now.
Do what you can, go as
far as you can, and do
the best you can right
now — at this moment.

DATE

STRENGTH
& FLEXIBILITY

ENDURANCE

COORDINATION
& BALANCE

CHALLENGES

MIND & SPIRIT

DATE

STRENGTH
& FLEXIBILITY

ENDURANCE

COORDINATION
& BALANCE

When you reach a point
of understanding and
acceptance of your weak
areas, you can go to
work on improving them.
Push yourself to improve
and progress each and
every time you perform
your Pilates routine.

CHALLENGES

MIND & SPIRIT

DATE

When the strength of
the powerhouse can
adequately support the
spine, we begin to strike
a balance physically.
Along with physical
balance, we reap the re-
wards of balance in many
other areas of our life.

STRENGTH
& FLEXIBILITY

ENDURANCE

COORDINATION
& BALANCE

CHALLENGES

MIND & SPIRIT

DATE

STRENGTH & FLEXIBILITY

ENDURANCE

COORDINATION & BALANCE

When you can physically
conquer the limitations
of your body, everything
in your life can get just
a little bit easier.

CHALLENGES

MIND & SPIRIT

DATE

STRENGTH
& FLEXIBILITY

ENDURANCE

COORDINATION
& BALANCE

CHALLENGES

MIND & SPIRIT

DATE

STRENGTH
& FLEXIBILITY

ENDURANCE

COORDINATION
& BALANCE

With each victory, we
encourage ourselves
to go further. With
progress comes a sense
of empowerment.

CHALLENGES

MIND & SPIRIT

DATE

Pilates will help you
to feel more confident.
It will help you to feel
prepared to take on any
challenge and it will
help to reduce your
stress level.

STRENGTH
& FLEXIBILITY

ENDURANCE

COORDINATION
& BALANCE

CHALLENGES

MIND & SPIRIT

DATE

STRENGTH
& FLEXIBILITY

ENDURANCE

COORDINATION
& BALANCE

CHALLENGES

The physical demands of
your routine will enable
you to feel a very deep
sense of relaxation and
have a tangible sense
that your daily stress is
slipping away effortlessly.

MIND & SPIRIT

DATE

STRENGTH & FLEXIBILITY

ENDURANCE

COORDINATION & BALANCE

CHALLENGES

MIND & SPIRIT

DATE

STRENGTH
& FLEXIBILITY

Pilates will help you
to be in the present,
and enable you to have
much more quality in
your quality time.

ENDURANCE

COORDINATION
& BALANCE

CHALLENGES

MIND & SPIRIT

DATE

STRENGTH
& FLEXIBILITY

ENDURANCE

COORDINATION
& BALANCE

CHALLENGES

It stands to reason that
anything operates better
when it's operated from
its center. So it is with
your body and in your
life. Pilates will allow you
to develop that center.

MIND & SPIRIT

DATE

STRENGTH & FLEXIBILITY

ENDURANCE

Pilates clears your mind,
and it allows you to be
centered and grounded,
so that you are more
effective and clear.

COORDINATION & BALANCE

CHALLENGES

MIND & SPIRIT

DATE

STRENGTH
& FLEXIBILITY

ENDURANCE

COORDINATION
& BALANCE

CHALLENGES

MIND & SPIRIT

DATE

STRENGTH
& FLEXIBILITY

ENDURANCE

COORDINATION
& BALANCE

Pilates can give you
a mildly intoxicating,
euphoric feeling. It is
very addicting. You'll
need it and crave it.
You'll find a way to
squeeze Pilates into
your busy schedule.

CHALLENGES

MIND & SPIRIT

DATE

Nature likes nothing
more than symmetry,
and when we achieve
physical symmetry
we become more
beautiful in the eyes
of the beholder.

STRENGTH
& FLEXIBILITY

ENDURANCE

COORDINATION
& BALANCE

CHALLENGES

MIND & SPIRIT

DATE

STRENGTH & FLEXIBILITY

ENDURANCE

COORDINATION & BALANCE

CHALLENGES

MIND & SPIRIT

"Pilates has changed
my body and made
me feel great."
Jamie Lee Curtis

DATE

STRENGTH
& FLEXIBILITY

ENDURANCE

COORDINATION
& BALANCE

CHALLENGES

MIND & SPIRIT

DATE

STRENGTH & FLEXIBILITY

ENDURANCE

Having balance in our
lives gives our life quality.
We find the room, and
more importantly, the
time to do everything
that we enjoy.

COORDINATION & BALANCE

CHALLENGES

MIND & SPIRIT

DATE

STRENGTH & FLEXIBILITY

ENDURANCE

When we live in the
moment, we are not
ruled by our past, nor
are we looking past
the here-and-now for
what is coming next.
We take it all in stride.

COORDINATION & BALANCE

CHALLENGES

MIND & SPIRIT

DATE

STRENGTH
& FLEXIBILITY

ENDURANCE

COORDINATION
& BALANCE

CHALLENGES

MIND & SPIRIT

DATE

STRENGTH & FLEXIBILITY

ENDURANCE

Being centered helps us
to be emotionally avail-
able, to be mentally
clear, to be capable of
accepting challenges,
to become more intuitive
and perceptive, and able
to achieve our potential.

COORDINATION & BALANCE

CHALLENGES

MIND & SPIRIT

DATE

STRENGTH
& FLEXIBILITY

ENDURANCE

COORDINATION
& BALANCE

Being present helps us
to be better listeners,
to have a deeper under-
standing of our present
situation and surround-
ings. We are better
spouses, better parents,
better friends, and better
people when we are
really, truly present.

CHALLENGES

MIND & SPIRIT

DATE

STRENGTH
& FLEXIBILITY

ENDURANCE

COORDINATION
& BALANCE

CHALLENGES

MIND & SPIRIT

DATE

STRENGTH
& FLEXIBILITY

ENDURANCE

COORDINATION
& BALANCE

CHALLENGES

It is the precise control
that you will demand
of your body that will
magically free your
mind up.

MIND & SPIRIT

The mental benefits of
Pilates are proportionate
to the quality of your
movement. Quality of
movement incorporates
being in control, being
aware of everything
going on inside of your
body and being keenly
aware of where you are.

STRENGTH
& FLEXIBILITY

ENDURANCE

COORDINATION
& BALANCE

CHALLENGES

MIND & SPIRIT

DATE

STRENGTH & FLEXIBILITY

ENDURANCE

COORDINATION & BALANCE

You will enhance the quality of your movement as you concentrate on how each movement flows into the next. Think of your routine as a perfectly choreographed dance piece and strive to make smooth transitions.

CHALLENGES

MIND & SPIRIT

STRENGTH
& FLEXIBILITY

ENDURANCE

COORDINATION
& BALANCE

CHALLENGES

MIND & SPIRIT

DATE

STRENGTH & FLEXIBILITY

ENDURANCE

COORDINATION & BALANCE

CHALLENGES

MIND & SPIRIT

You must not be overly
critical of your abilities.
Don't worry about
doing something wrong,
just move through the
routine. If you have to
make little mistakes,
you make little mistakes.

DATE

It's the continuation and the fluidity of the movement that's the most important thing in Pilates. This is the key to incorporating quality into the movement.

STRENGTH & FLEXIBILITY

ENDURANCE

COORDINATION & BALANCE

CHALLENGES

MIND & SPIRIT

DATE

STRENGTH
& FLEXIBILITY

ENDURANCE

COORDINATION
& BALANCE

CHALLENGES

MIND & SPIRIT

DATE

Experience your body as
one whole mechanism.
When all the moving
parts of your mechanism
are working together
as one, it is the most
amazing and wondrous
experience.

STRENGTH
& FLEXIBILITY

ENDURANCE

COORDINATION
& BALANCE

CHALLENGES

MIND & SPIRIT

DATE

STRENGTH
& FLEXIBILITY

ENDURANCE

COORDINATION
& BALANCE

CHALLENGES

"Pilates is the
face-lift of the
new millennium."
Dixie Carter

MIND & SPIRIT

DATE _____

STRENGTH
& FLEXIBILITY

ENDURANCE

COORDINATION
& BALANCE

CHALLENGES

MIND & SPIRIT

DATE

When you are at peace
with yourself and when
your entire body is work-
ing in harmony you will
experience joy. That is
the joy of movement.

When we have an injury
that prevents us from
doing what we normally
do or what we want
to do, it is defeating.
Mentally and physically
it debilitates us. If you
give into it, you give in
to defeat.

STRENGTH & FLEXIBILITY

ENDURANCE

COORDINATION & BALANCE

CHALLENGES

MIND & SPIRIT

DATE

STRENGTH & FLEXIBILITY

ENDURANCE

COORDINATION & BALANCE

CHALLENGES

When we are centered
mentally, we have the
strength to stand up for
ourselves, because we
are dealing from the
truest and purest portion
of our being.

MIND & SPIRIT

DATE

STRENGTH
& FLEXIBILITY

ENDURANCE

COORDINATION
& BALANCE

CHALLENGES

MIND & SPIRIT

DATE

STRENGTH & FLEXIBILITY

ENDURANCE

COORDINATION & BALANCE

CHALLENGES

MIND & SPIRIT

You cannot and must not let your pain defeat you. If you must modify a movement to get through it, do so. When you can work through your pain, you can come out on the other side. That is a victory.

DATE

You are never too old
to be active. Aside from
the physical benefits,
Pilates will help you
hone your memory, and
will give you an overall
sense of well being.

STRENGTH
& FLEXIBILITY

ENDURANCE

COORDINATION
& BALANCE

CHALLENGES

MIND & SPIRIT

DATE

STRENGTH
& FLEXIBILITY

ENDURANCE

Joseph Pilates referred
to the powerhouse as
"the girdle of strength."

COORDINATION
& BALANCE

CHALLENGES

MIND & SPIRIT

DATE

STRENGTH
& FLEXIBILITY

ENDURANCE

COORDINATION
& BALANCE

CHALLENGES

MIND & SPIRIT

DATE

STRENGTH & FLEXIBILITY

ENDURANCE

When doing Pilates,
concentrate on your
breath and make certain
to exhale completely.
You must really wring
out your lungs when
you exhale. Expel all
of that contaminated
air inside of you and
breathe in fresh air to
rejuvenate the body.

COORDINATION & BALANCE

CHALLENGES

MIND & SPIRIT

DATE

STRENGTH
& FLEXIBILITY

ENDURANCE

COORDINATION
& BALANCE

CHALLENGES

Pilates represents a shift
in orientation. Pilates
represents the orienta-
tion of healing the body
and preventing injury.

MIND & SPIRIT

DATE

STRENGTH
& FLEXIBILITY

ENDURANCE

COORDINATION
& BALANCE

CHALLENGES

MIND & SPIRIT

The powerhouse is
key to your physical
trans-formation, but
it is also essential in
developing a higher,
more enlightened self.

DATE

MIND & SPIRIT

CHALLENGES

COORDINATION
& BALANCE

ENDURANCE

STRENGTH
& FLEXIBILITY

DATE

STRENGTH
& FLEXIBILITY

ENDURANCE

COORDINATION
& BALANCE

CHALLENGES

MIND & SPIRIT

In Pilates, you will
immediately notice that
your posture and the
way you carry yourself
will be much improved
and this may feel very
new and different to you.
In one month's time
those around you will
be certain that you are
changing.

DATE

One of the many benefits
the Pilates method of
body conditioning offers
is to vastly improve our
movement consciousness
— an awareness of
where you are in time
and space.

STRENGTH
& FLEXIBILITY

ENDURANCE

COORDINATION
& BALANCE

CHALLENGES

MIND & SPIRIT

DATE

STRENGTH
& FLEXIBILITY

ENDURANCE

It is from the reliance
upon and strengthening
of the powerhouse that
you will derive all of the
physical, mental, and
spiritual benefits of this
form of exercise.

COORDINATION
& BALANCE

CHALLENGES

MIND & SPIRIT

DATE

STRENGTH
& FLEXIBILITY

ENDURANCE

COORDINATION
& BALANCE

CHALLENGES

MIND & SPIRIT

DATE

STRENGTH
& FLEXIBILITY

ENDURANCE

COORDINATION
& BALANCE

CHALLENGES

In Pilates, all movement
emanates from the
powerhouse — the place
that connects the stom-
ach with the spine with
the buttocks. From this
place you become very
aware of movement, and
of how that center sup-
ports movement in a
very positive way.

MIND & SPIRIT

DATE

In Pilates, we work inside the frame of the body. When you are standing, your legs should be underneath your hips; your arms should be underneath your shoulders. Your shoulders and hips should "frame" your body.

STRENGTH & FLEXIBILITY

ENDURANCE

COORDINATION & BALANCE

CHALLENGES

MIND & SPIRIT

DATE

The balance and alignment of your body are the keys to preventing injury. When your washing machine is out of balance, you can hear it clanking all through the house. So it is with your body.

ENDURANCE

COORDINATION & BALANCE

CHALLENGES

MIND & SPIRIT

DATE

STRENGTH
& FLEXIBILITY

ENDURANCE

COORDINATION
& BALANCE

CHALLENGES

MIND & SPIRIT

DATE

In Pilates, all movements are generated by your powerhouse. Whenever you do an exercise, movement and control over that movement is always initiated by breathing into and pushing from the powerhouse.

DATE

Pilates will help you to
balance the body, but
you must be mindful
of working evenly.
If you have one side
that is stronger than
the other, then you
want to work harder
on the weaker side.

STRENGTH
& FLEXIBILITY

ENDURANCE

COORDINATION
& BALANCE

CHALLENGES

MIND & SPIRIT

DATE

STRENGTH
& FLEXIBILITY

ENDURANCE

COORDINATION
& BALANCE

CHALLENGES

"The Pilates tech-
nique has proven to
be the absolute best
workout for my body,
mind and soul."
Elizabeth Berkley

MIND & SPIRIT

DATE

MIND & SPIRIT

CHALLENGES

COORDINATION
& BALANCE

ENDURANCE

STRENGTH
& FLEXIBILITY

DATE

STRENGTH & FLEXIBILITY

ENDURANCE

COORDINATION & BALANCE

CHALLENGES

MIND & SPIRIT

In balancing your body, you are doing something extraordinarily healthy for yourself. When you are in balance, you are in harmony with yourself and the world around you.

DATE

Being centered, or
striking a balance be-
tween the mind and
the body, is a place that
we want to occupy more
and more frequently.
It is much like a muscle
that we want to develop.

STRENGTH
& FLEXIBILITY

ENDURANCE

COORDINATION
& BALANCE

CHALLENGES

MIND & SPIRIT

DATE

STRENGTH & FLEXIBILITY

ENDURANCE

COORDINATION & BALANCE

With Pilates your body is able to work more efficiently and at a higher level. When operating on this higher level, you can live your life passionately and euphorically.

CHALLENGES

MIND & SPIRIT

DATE

Pilates brings the body
into a state of harmony,
so that everything is
working together as
one unit. That is the joy
of movement.

STRENGTH
& FLEXIBILITY

ENDURANCE

COORDINATION
& BALANCE

CHALLENGES

MIND & SPIRIT

DATE

STRENGTH
& FLEXIBILITY

ENDURANCE

COORDINATION
& BALANCE

CHALLENGES

MIND & SPIRIT

DATE

When you inhale,
breathe into the back in
the area that expands
the small ribs. This form
of deep breathing allows
us to bend and move
without restricting the
amount of oxygen that
we are taking in.

STRENGTH & FLEXIBILITY

ENDURANCE

COORDINATION & BALANCE

CHALLENGES

MIND & SPIRIT

DATE

STRENGTH
& FLEXIBILITY

ENDURANCE

COORDINATION
& BALANCE

CHALLENGES

With Pilates, each move-
ment is tied to a specific
manner of breathing.
Breath allows oxygen
to nourish the muscles
being utilized, and to
release an array of non-
beneficial chemicals
stored in the muscles.

MIND & SPIRIT

DATE

It is important to drink a
lot of water — a marked
increase in intake —
when you are working
out. Hydrating the body
effectively can offset
soreness.

STRENGTH
& FLEXIBILITY

ENDURANCE

COORDINATION
& BALANCE

CHALLENGES

MIND & SPIRIT

DATE

STRENGTH
& FLEXIBILITY

ENDURANCE

COORDINATION
& BALANCE

CHALLENGES

MIND & SPIRIT

DATE

With Pilates, it is the involvement of the entire body that helps to relieve tension in the body. After you finish your routine you will notice that you have eliminated stress significantly on both the physical and mental levels.

STRENGTH & FLEXIBILITY

ENDURANCE

COORDINATION & BALANCE

CHALLENGES

MIND & SPIRIT

DATE

STRENGTH
& FLEXIBILITY

ENDURANCE

COORDINATION
& BALANCE

Our goal is to have the
mental and physical
working in conjunction
with one another —
a mind/body connection.

CHALLENGES

MIND & SPIRIT

DATE

As our ability to concentrate on a specific area of the body improves, we dramatically enhance the quality of our movement.

STRENGTH & FLEXIBILITY

ENDURANCE

COORDINATION & BALANCE

CHALLENGES

MIND & SPIRIT

DATE

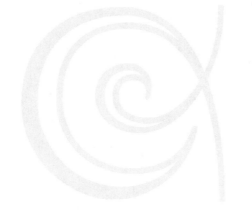

STRENGTH & FLEXIBILITY

ENDURANCE

COORDINATION & BALANCE

CHALLENGES

MIND & SPIRIT

DATE _____

STRENGTH
& FLEXIBILITY

ENDURANCE

COORDINATION
& BALANCE

CHALLENGES

The quality of being
graceful while you
perform this movement
stems from the fluidity
of one movement
seamlessly blending
into the next.

MIND & SPIRIT

DATE

STRENGTH
& FLEXIBILITY

ENDURANCE

"Pilates has healed
my hamstring,
increased my flexi-
bility and overall
strength."
Jasmine Guy

COORDINATION
& BALANCE

CHALLENGES

MIND & SPIRIT

DATE

STRENGTH
& FLEXIBILITY

ENDURANCE

COORDINATION
& BALANCE

CHALLENGES

MIND & SPIRIT

DATE

STRENGTH & FLEXIBILITY

Each Pilates exercise has a specific point at which it begins, and a place where it ends. It is your task to make these places blend into each other, to be unrecogniz- able points of reference within the whole.

ENDURANCE

COORDINATION & BALANCE

CHALLENGES

MIND & SPIRIT

DATE

An instruction to "hold" an exercise for a certain number of counts is not a place to stop, but rather a place where a stretch or movement continues, however un-recognizable it may be to an outside observer.

STRENGTH & FLEXIBILITY

ENDURANCE

COORDINATION & BALANCE

CHALLENGES

MIND & SPIRIT

DATE

STRENGTH
& FLEXIBILITY

ENDURANCE

COORDINATION
& BALANCE

CHALLENGES

As you strengthen your
powerhouse, you will,
in fact, strengthen every
aspect of your life. It
allows for possibility to
enter into your mind and
your spirit and your life.

MIND & SPIRIT

DATE

Each exercise leads to
the next. There is really
no time when your move-
ment stops. The end of
one movement is just the
beginning of another.

STRENGTH
& FLEXIBILITY

ENDURANCE

COORDINATION
& BALANCE

CHALLENGES

MIND & SPIRIT

DATE

DATE

Each Pilates exercise
links breathing with
strengthening and
stretching. Each move-
ment is designed to
scientifically oxygenate,
then stretch, then
strengthen, and then
re-stretch a particular
muscle group.

STRENGTH
& FLEXIBILITY

ENDURANCE

COORDINATION
& BALANCE

CHALLENGES

MIND & SPIRIT

DATE

STRENGTH
& FLEXIBILITY

ENDURANCE

COORDINATION
& BALANCE

When we are mindful
of our movement, we
can employ both the
brain and the body to
work harmoniously
and effectively.

CHALLENGES

MIND & SPIRIT

DATE

STRENGTH
& FLEXIBILITY

ENDURANCE

COORDINATION
& BALANCE

CHALLENGES

MIND & SPIRIT

DATE

STRENGTH & FLEXIBILITY

ENDURANCE

The premise of Pilates is
to strengthen smaller
muscle groups to sup-
port larger muscles.

COORDINATION & BALANCE

CHALLENGES

MIND & SPIRIT

DATE

As we focus on pulling
in the powerhouse,
the place in our gut that
links the stomach with
the lower back with the
butt, we can instantly
feel a lengthening sen-
sation in the lower back.

STRENGTH
& FLEXIBILITY

ENDURANCE

COORDINATION
& BALANCE

CHALLENGES

MIND & SPIRIT

DATE

STRENGTH
& FLEXIBILITY

ENDURANCE

Mentally, the control
that you exert over your
powerhouse translates
into a calm and clarity,
from which you can take
life's challenges and deal
with them appropriately.

COORDINATION
& BALANCE

CHALLENGES

MIND & SPIRIT

DATE

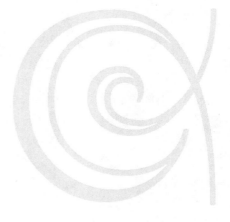

STRENGTH & FLEXIBILITY

ENDURANCE

COORDINATION & BALANCE

CHALLENGES

MIND & SPIRIT

DATE

STRENGTH & FLEXIBILITY

ENDURANCE

The more you concentrate on your body parts working in harmony with one another, the straighter your spine becomes.

COORDINATION & BALANCE

CHALLENGES

MIND & SPIRIT

DATE

STRENGTH
& FLEXIBILITY

ENDURANCE

The key to Pilates is to
pull your powerhouse
toward your spine.

COORDINATION
& BALANCE

CHALLENGES

MIND & SPIRIT

DATE

STRENGTH & FLEXIBILITY

ENDURANCE

COORDINATION & BALANCE

CHALLENGES

MIND & SPIRIT

If you can learn to control your powerhouse, and initiate movement from this place, a whole new world of physical movement will be revealed to you.

DATE

Appendix

beginner routine	intermediate routine	advanced routine	
The Hundred	The Hundred	The Hundred	Teaser #2
Roll-Ups	Roll-Ups	Roll-Ups	Teaser #3
Single Leg Circles	Single Leg Circles	Single Leg Circles	Single Leg Teaser
Rolling Like a Ball	Rolling Like a Ball	Rolling Like a Ball	Hip Circles
Single Leg Stretch	Single Leg Stretch	Roll-Over	Can-Can
Double Leg Stretch	Double Leg Stretch	Single Leg Stretch	Kneeling Side Kicks
Single Straight Leg	Single Straight Leg	Double Leg Stretch	The Mermaid
Double Straight Leg	Double Straight Leg	Single Straight Leg	Scissors
Spine Stretch Forward	The Criss-Cross	Double Straight Leg	Bicycle
The Saw	Spine Stretch Forward	The Criss-Cross	Shoulder Bridge
Neck Roll	Corkscrew	Spine Stretch Forward	Leg Pull Down
Single Leg Kick	The Saw	Corkscrew	Leg Pull Up
Little Piece of Heaven	Open Leg Rocker	The Saw	Boomerang
Total Butt Workout	Neck Roll	Open Leg Rocker	The Seal
Closing	Single Leg Kick	Neck Roll	Push-Ups
	Double Leg Kick	Single Leg Kick	Total Butt Workout
	Swimming	Double Leg Kick	Closing
	Little Piece of Heaven	Swimming	
	Neck Pull	Little Piece of Heaven	
	Side Kick Series	Neck Pull	
	Teaser #1	Spine Twist	
	The Seal	The Jackknife	
	Total Butt Workout	Side Kick Series	
	Closing	Teaser #1	